5-Minute Mindfulness

5-Minute Mindfulness

Quick Guides to a Calmer You

B. Vincent

QuantumQuill Press

Contents

Chapter 1: Introduction to Mindfulness

What is Mindfulness?

In our fast-paced, digitally pushed world, the thinking of mindfulness has emerged as a beacon of serenity amidst the chaos. But what precisely is mindfulness, and the place does it originate? At its core, mindfulness is the exercise of deliberately paying interest to the current second besides judgment. It attracts upon historical Buddhist principles, in particular these observed in Vipassana and Zen traditions, which emphasize cognizance and acceptance of truth as it unfolds.

Mindfulness invitations us to anchor our cognizance in the right here and now, turning into attuned to our thoughts, feelings, bodily sensations, and the surroundings round us. Rather than living on the previous or fretting about the future, mindfulness encourages us to entirely inhabit the present, embracing every second with openness and curiosity.

In our cutting-edge context, mindfulness has garnered sizable consciousness for its profound advantages to mental, emotional, and bodily well-being. From lowering stress and nervousness to improving focal point and emotional resilience, the exercise of mindfulness gives a holistic method to cultivating internal peace and contentment.

As we embark on this ride into the coronary heart of mindfulness, let us discover its essence, its relevance in our lives today, and the transformative energy it holds for these who dare to embark upon its path.

Benefits of Practicing Mindfulness

Within the tumultuous currents of contemporary existence, the exercise of mindfulness serves as a steadfast anchor, providing refuge amidst life's storms. As we delve deeper into the nation-states of mindfulness, it turns into evident that its rewards prolong a ways past the confines of fleeting moments. Let us embark on a trip to find the manifold advantages that look forward to these who select to include mindfulness in their day by day lives.

Stress Reduction: In the hustle and bustle of our stressful lives, stress regularly reigns as an unwelcome companion. However, via the exercise of mindfulness, we find out a mighty antidote to the perils of stress. By cultivating present-moment focus and fostering a nonjudgmental mind-set toward our experiences, we research to navigate life's challenges with grace and equanimity.

Improved Focus and Concentration: In an age characterized by way of consistent distractions and statistics overload, preserving focal point can experience like an elusive feat. Yet, mindfulness provides a sanctuary of readability amidst the chaos. By honing our potential to direct our interest to the existing moment, we domesticate a sharpened center of attention and heightened concentration, enabling us to interact greater wholly with the duties at hand.

Enhanced Emotional Regulation: Emotions, like turbulent waves, frequently threaten to crush us, leaving us feeling adrift in a sea of uncertainty. However, thru the exercise of mindfulness, we obtain useful equipment for navigating the depths of our emotional landscape. By staring at our ideas and emotions with compassionate curiosity, as a substitute than reacting impulsively, we boost larger emotional talent and resilience.

Better Relationships: At the coronary heart of our human trip lies the tricky internet of relationships that bind us together. Yet, amidst the complexities of interpersonal dynamics, misunderstandings and conflicts can occur all too easily. Through the lens of mindfulness, however, we find out a pathway to deeper connection and empathy. By cultivating present-moment recognition and lively listening, we foster extra significant and real relationships with others.

Physical Health Benefits: The mind-body connection lies at the core of mindfulness, underscoring the profound affect that our intellectual nation can have on our bodily well-being. Numerous research have highlighted the myriad fitness advantages related with mindfulness practice, consisting of decreased blood pressure, extended immune function, and superior ache management. By nurturing our internal panorama thru mindfulness, we pave the way for increased vitality and vitality.

As we replicate upon these transformative benefits, let us include the exercise of mindfulness with open hearts and minds, understanding that the experience in the direction of increased well-being starts with a single breath.

Myths and Misconceptions about Mindfulness

In the good sized panorama of human understanding, myths and misconceptions frequently shroud the truth, obscuring readability and inviting confusion. As we embark on our exploration of mindfulness, it is imperative to dispel these veils of misinformation, illuminating the direction with the mild of reality and understanding. Let us navigate thru the murky waters of misconception, unveiling the essence of mindfulness that lies beneath.

Common Misunderstandings: Like whispers carried by way of the wind, myths about mindfulness permeate our collective consciousness, clouding our appreciation with falsehoods and half-truths. One time-honored false impression suggests that mindfulness is synonymous with leisure or escapism, portraying it as a mere device for transient comfort from life's challenges. However, mindfulness transcends the realm of short-term relaxation, inviting us to embody the full spectrum of our human journey with readability and presence.

Dispelling Misconceptions: To unravel the tangled net of misunderstanding, we have to shine the mild of fact upon its threads, revealing the inherent knowledge of mindfulness. Contrary to famous belief, mindfulness does now not require us to suppress or get rid of our ideas and emotions. Instead, it invitations us to examine them with compassionate awareness, acknowledging their presence besides judgment or attachment. By cultivating this non-judgmental stance, we research to navigate the ebb and go with the flow of our internal panorama with grace and equanimity.

As we navigate the labyrinth of misconception, let us strategy mindfulness with open hearts and open minds, understanding that genuine grasp arises now not from blind acceptance of preconceived notions, however from the willingness to question, explore, and find out the fact for ourselves.

How Mindfulness Works

In the tricky dance of existence, the exercise of mindfulness serves as a guiding light, illuminating the course to internal peace and clarity. But how does mindfulness work its transformative magic upon the human psyche? Let us embark on a trip of exploration, delving into the internal workings of mindfulness and uncovering the profound insights it holds.

Understanding the Mechanism: At its essence, mindfulness entails the cultivation of present-moment awareness, inviting us to anchor our interest in the right here and now. Through practices such as meditation, breath awareness, and physique scanning, we teach our minds to have a look at the drift of thoughts, emotions, and sensations with unbiased curiosity. By growing this potential for nonjudgmental observation, we domesticate a deeper appreciation of ourselves and the world round us.

Neuroscience Behind Mindfulness: As contemporary science delves deeper into the mysteries of the mind, researchers have begun to unravel the neural mechanisms underlying mindfulness practice. Neuroimaging research have published that normal mindfulness exercise can lead to structural modifications in the brain, specifically in areas related with attention, emotion regulation, and self-awareness. Moreover, mindfulness has been proven to modulate pastime in the amygdala, the brain's concern center, lowering reactivity to stress and improving emotional resilience.

As we peer under the floor of mindfulness, we find out a wealthy tapestry of insights drawn from each historical knowledge traditions and present day scientific inquiry. By appreciation the mechanisms via which mindfulness exerts its transformative influence, we empower ourselves to embark on a trip of self-discovery and internal transformation with readability and confidence.

Setting Intentions for Your Mindfulness Practice

In the massive expanse of human experience, intention serves as a guiding star, illuminating the route to purposeful dwelling and significant transformation. As we embark on our experience into the coronary heart of mindfulness, it is critical to set clear intentions that will information and preserve our practice. Let us embark on a voyage of self-discovery and internal exploration, anchoring ourselves in the fertile soil of intentionality.

Clarifying Goals: Like a captain charting a path throughout uncharted waters, putting clear dreams serves as the compass that courses our trip into mindfulness. Take a second to replicate on what you hope to attain thru your practice. Whether it is lowering stress, cultivating internal peace, or deepening self-awareness, articulating your intentions with readability and specificity empowers you to navigate the complexities of the internal panorama with motive and direction.

Commitment to the Journey: In the face of life's myriad distractions and challenges, dedication serves as the bedrock upon which our mindfulness exercise is built. Cultivate a spirit of dedication and perseverance, recognizing that genuine transformation unfolds progressively over time. Just as a gardener tends to their backyard with endurance and care, nurture your mindfulness exercise with unwavering commitment, understanding that every second of aware cognizance brings you one step nearer to the success of your intentions.

As you embark on this sacred trip of self-discovery and internal transformation, let your intentions serve as beacons of light, guiding you via the turbulent waters of the thought with grace and steadfastness. With every breath, every second of conscious awareness, you step ever nearer to realizing the fullness of your being and embracing the countless manageable that lies within.

{ **2** }

Chapter 2: 5-Minute Mindfulness Exercises

Breath Awareness

In the rush of each day life, amidst the whirlwind of obligations and distractions, the breath stands as an ever-present anchor, a steadfast accomplice inviting us returned to the existing moment. In the exercise of breath awareness, we harness the electricity of the breath as a gateway to mindfulness, a doorway thru which we may also enter into the depths of our being.

Simple Breathing Exercises: At its essence, breath recognition starts off evolved with a return to the breath itself, the rhythmic ebb and glide that sustains us in each moment. Through easy respiratory exercises, such as deep stomach respiratory or aware breathing, we attune our consciousness to the sensations of the breath as it strikes in and out of the body. With every inhalation and exhalation, we domesticate a experience of groundedness and presence, anchoring ourselves in the right here and now.

Connecting with the Present Moment: As we deepen into the exercise of breath awareness, we commence to unravel the elaborate tapestry of our internal experience, looking at the sensations, thoughts, and feelings that occur with every breath. With mild curiosity and nonjudgmental awareness, we witness the ceaseless dance of the breath, recognizing it as a reflect reflecting the ever-changing panorama of our minds and bodies.

In the sanctuary of breath awareness, we locate solace amidst the chaos, a refuge of calm amidst the storm. Through the easy act of returning to the breath, once more and again, we find out a profound feel of peace and readability that transcends the turbulence of the exterior world. In the rhythm of our breath, we reclaim our inherent birthright to dwell in the timeless realm of the existing moment, the place proper freedom and achievement await.

Body Scan

In the labyrinth of the human experience, the physique serves as a sacred vessel, a repository of knowledge and perception ready to be discovered. Through the exercise of the physique scan, we embark on a experience of self-exploration, delving into the depths of our bodily being with aware recognition and compassionate presence.

Progressive Relaxation: At the coronary heart of the physique scan lies the artwork of revolutionary relaxation, a mild but effective approach for releasing anxiety and merchandising deep relaxation. As we systematically scan thru every phase of the body, from head to toe, we invite recognition to penetrate deeply into the muscles, bones, and tissues, bringing interest to any areas of tightness or discomfort. With every breath, every second of conscious attention, we provide ourselves the present of relaxation, permitting the physique to soften and lay down into a nation of profound ease.

Releasing Tension: In the crucible of current life, the physique frequently bears the brunt of our accrued stress and tension, manifesting as tightness, stiffness, or discomfort. Through the exercise of the physique scan, we domesticate an intimate cognizance of these bodily sensations, getting to know to meet them with kindness and compassion alternatively than resistance or judgment. By bringing aware interest to areas of tension, we create house for recovery and release, permitting the physique to unwind and return to a country of equilibrium.

As we trip deeper into the geographical regions of the physique scan, we find out a profound feel of connection and integration, a merging of mind, body, and spirit into a harmonious whole. In the sanctuary of our personal bodies, we discover a refuge of peace and presence, a sacred temple the place the mild of consciousness illuminates the course to recovery and wholeness.

Observing Thoughts and Emotions

In the giant panorama of the mind, ideas and feelings swirl like leaves caught in a mild breeze, ephemeral but profoundly impactful. Through the exercise of looking at ideas and feelings with aware awareness, we embark on a experience of self-discovery and internal transformation, cultivating a spacious and compassionate relationship with the ever-changing panorama of our internal world.

Witnessing Thoughts Without Judgment: In the tumult of the mind, ideas occur like waves upon the floor of the ocean, fleeting and transient. Yet, all too often, we end up entangled in the currents of our very own thoughts, swept away by means of the tide of rumination and worry. Through the exercise of mindfulness, we research to step again from the incessant chatter of the mind, staring at our ideas with spacious focus and nonjudgmental curiosity. By cultivating this stance of indifferent observation, we create house for perception and grasp to arise, untethered via the grip of routine patterns of thought.

Cultivating Emotional Resilience: Emotions, like climate patterns, ebb and waft with the rhythm of life, carrying us on a ride of highs and lows, joys and sorrows. Yet, amidst the tempest of our emotional landscape, lies the possibility for increase and transformation. Through the exercise of mindfulness, we analyze to greet our feelings with open arms, embracing them as messengers bearing treasured insights about our innermost wishes and fears. By cultivating a compassionate mindset in the direction of our emotions, we boost larger emotional resilience, mastering to trip the waves of ride with grace and equanimity.

As we trip deeper into the geographical regions of staring at ideas and emotions, we find out a profound experience of freedom and empowerment, a liberation from the shackles of recurring re-activity and unconscious conditioning. In the spacious expanse of aware awareness, we discover refuge amidst the turbulence of the mind, embracing every notion and emotion as a treasured present on the direction to self-discovery and awakening.

Gratitude Practice

In the hustle and bustle of cutting-edge life, amidst the cease-less cacophony of needs and distractions, the exercise of gratitude stands as a beacon of light, illuminating the route to internal peace and contentment. Through the cultivation of gratitude, we awaken to the abundance that surrounds us, inviting pleasure and achieve-ment into our hearts with every second of aware awareness.

Focusing on Appreciation: At its core, gratitude is a exercise of transferring our center of attention from what is missing to what is present, from shortage to abundance. Through the exercise of gratitude, we educate our minds to apprehend and recognize the myriad advantages that grace our lives every day, from the easy pleasures of a heat cup of tea to the profound splendor of a sun-down portray the sky in shades of gold and crimson. By anchoring our cognizance in the existing second and opening our hearts to the richness of our experience, we domesticate a deep feel of grasp for the many presents that lifestyles has to offer.

Shifting Perspective: In the crucible of adversity, the exercise of gratitude serves as a effective antidote to despair, supplying solace and power in the face of life's challenges. By reframing our perceptions and focusing on the benefits that occur even in the midst of difficulty, we find out resilience and grace past measure. Through the lens of gratitude, each impediment will become an probability for growth, each and every setback a stepping stone on the direction to higher knowledge and understanding.

As we trip deeper into the nation-states of gratitude practice, we find out a profound feel of interconnectedness and belonging, a consciousness that we are woven into the cloth of the universe itself. In the embody of gratitude, we discover refuge amidst the uncertainties of life, anchoring ourselves in the timeless reality that love and abundance abound, ready patiently for us to open our hearts and obtain their boundless blessings.

Loving-Kindness Meditation

In the labyrinth of the human heart, love stands as the remaining guiding force, illuminating the course to healing, connection, and wholeness. Through the exercise of loving-kindness meditation, we embark on a ride of profound self-discovery and internal transformation, cultivating boundless compassion and unconditional love for ourselves and all beings.

Cultivating Compassion: At its essence, loving-kindness meditation is a exercise of extending goodwill and benevolence closer to ourselves and others. Through a collection of guided phrases or visualizations, we deliberately domesticate emotions of kindness, compassion, and love, radiating these traits outwards like rays of sunshine, touching the hearts of all beings with heat and tenderness. By nurturing a experience of deep care and subject for the well-being of ourselves and others, we awaken to the intercon-nectedness of all existence and the inherent worthiness of each and every being.

Spreading Positivity Towards Oneself and Others: In the cruci-ble of self-judgment and criticism, the exercise of loving-kindness gives a balm of restoration and acceptance, inviting us to include ourselves with the identical unconditional love and compassion that we prolong to others. Through the exercise of loving-kindness meditation, we analyze to soften the harsh edges of self-doubt and self-criticism, cultivating a experience of deep self-acceptance and self-love that permeates each thing of our being. As we open our hearts to ourselves, we naturally prolong this equal love and kind-ness to others, developing ripples of positivity and goodwill that ripple outwards, touching the lives of all beings with grace and beauty.

As we trip deeper into the nation-states of loving-kindness meditation, we find out a profound experience of interconnected-ness and belonging, a focus that we are all threads in the tapestry of existence, woven collectively by using the bonds of love and compassion. In the include of loving-kindness, we discover refuge amidst the uncertainties of life, anchoring ourselves in the timeless reality that love is the closing recuperation force, uniting us all in a sacred dance of grace and beauty.

Chapter 3: Integrating Mindfulness into Daily Life

Mindful Eating

In the frenetic tempo of modern-day life, meal instances regularly come to be mere pit stops in the race of productivity, overshadowed through multitasking and senseless consumption. However, with the aid of infusing the exercise of mindfulness into our consuming habits, we can radically change these moments into possibilities for profound nourishment and presence.

Paying Attention to the Senses: Mindful ingesting starts with a return to the current moment, inviting us to have interaction wholly with the sensory journey of eating. As we sit down to a meal, we awaken our senses to the prosperous tapestry of colors, textures, and aromas earlier than us. With every bite, we get pleasure from the flavors dancing upon our style buds, relishing the nourishment that sustains our bodies and nourishes our souls. By paying interest to the sensations of starvation and fullness, we domesticate a deeper focus of our body's signals, honoring its knowledge and fostering a greater intuitive relationship with food.

Cultivating a Healthy Relationship with Food: Beyond nourishing our bodies, conscious ingesting presents a pathway to recuperation our relationship with meals and our bodies. Through the exercise of aware awareness, we domesticate a compassionate mindset in the direction of ourselves and our consuming habits, releasing judgments and expectations that may additionally have clouded our trip in the past. By drawing close every meal with curiosity and kindness, we create area for larger self-acceptance and self-care, nourishing now not solely our bodies however additionally our hearts and minds.

As we combine mindfulness into our consuming habits, we reclaim the sacredness of meal times, honoring the interconnectedness of food, body, and spirit. In the easy act of consuming with focus and gratitude, we find out a profound feel of nourishment and fulfillment, reconnecting with the inherent pleasure and abundance that lies inside every bite.

Mindful Movement

Amidst the hustle and bustle of current life, motion regularly turns into a capacity to an end, a hurried rush from one undertaking to the next, devoid of presence or purpose. Yet, with the aid of infusing the exercise of mindfulness into our movement, we can seriously change even the easiest moves into possibilities for profound focus and connection.

Incorporating Mindfulness into Physical Activities: Mindful motion invitations us to deliver our full interest and intention to each and every action, whether or not it be walking, stretching, or enticing in a formal workout routine. As we cross our bodies with awareness, we emerge as attuned to the sensations, rhythms, and nuances of movement, cultivating a deeper perception for the excellent vessel that consists of us via life. By honoring the existing second with every step and every breath, we invite a feel of ease and grace into our movements, fostering a harmonious union of body, mind, and spirit.

Yoga, Walking, and Other Exercises: Mindful motion encompasses a huge array of activities, from the mild flowing sequences of yoga to the rhythmic cadence of strolling meditation. Whether we are enticing in a formal exercise or virtually going about our every day activities, each motion provides an possibility to domesticate mindfulness and presence. By coming near every motion with intention and attention, we radically change workout from a chore into a sacred ritual, a get together of the body's innate knowledge and vitality.

As we combine mindfulness into our motion practices, we awaken to the profound interconnectedness of physique and mind, honoring the sacred dance of lifestyles unfolding inside and round us. In the mild rhythm of our breath and the fluidity of our movements, we find out a sanctuary of peace and presence, reconnecting with the timeless knowledge that resides at the coronary heart of our embodied existence.

Mindful Communication

In the symphony of human interaction, conversation serves as the melody that binds us together, weaving threads of connection and grasp amidst the cacophony of noise. Through the exercise of conscious communication, we embark on a experience of deep listening and real expression, fostering richer and extra significant connections with ourselves and others.

Listening with Full Attention: At the coronary heart of aware conversation lies the artwork of listening with presence and empathy, providing our full interest to the words, emotions, and nuances conveyed via others. Instead of certainly ready for our flip to speak, we domesticate a spacious consciousness that permits us to really hear and apprehend the messages being communicated, each verbally and nonverbally. By suspending judgment and tuning into the underlying wishes and intentions of the speaker, we create a protected and supportive house for genuine sharing and mutual grasp to flourish.

Responding Rather than Reacting: Mindful verbal exchange invitations us to reply to conditions with intention and discernment, alternatively than reacting impulsively from a vicinity of addiction or reactivity. By pausing to mirror on our ideas and thoughts earlier than speaking, we domesticate increased self-awareness and emotional intelligence, selecting our phrases and movements with care and compassion. In doing so, we honor the energy of our phrases to uplift and inspire, fostering harmony and connection in our relationships and communities.

As we combine conscious verbal exchange into our day by day interactions, we awaken to the transformative possible of our phrases and presence, recognizing that each and every alternate gives an possibility to domesticate larger understanding, empathy, and connection. In the sacred house of conscious communication, we co-create a world the place authenticity, respect, and compassion reign supreme, fostering a tradition of concord and belonging that reverberates at some stage in the tapestry of human experience.

Mindful Work

Amidst the hustle and bustle of the contemporary workplace, mindfulness provides a sanctuary of calm amidst the storm, a refuge of presence amidst the chaos. Through the exercise of mindfulness at work, we domesticate higher clarity, focus, and resilience, empowering ourselves to navigate the challenges of our expert lives with grace and equanimity.

Enhancing Productivity and Creativity: Mindfulness at work starts off evolved with a dedication to presence and intentionality in our every day duties and interactions. By bringing our full interest to the existing moment, we domesticate a heightened feel of center of attention and concentration, enabling us to work extra effectively and effectively. Moreover, with the aid of quieting the incessant chatter of the mind, we create house for creativity and innovation to flourish, tapping into the wellspring of notion that resides inside every of us.

Managing Workplace Stress: In the stress cooker of the present day workplace, stress frequently runs rampant, sapping our electricity and eroding our well-being. However, via the exercise of mindfulness, we can strengthen increased resilience in the face of adversity, mastering to reply to difficult conditions with calm and readability as an alternative than reactive panic. By cultivating a feel of spacious consciousness and self-compassion, we create a buffer towards the stresses and traces of the workday, fostering a feel of stability and well-being that permeates each and every thing of our expert lives.

As we combine mindfulness into our work routines, we find out a profound feel of empowerment and fulfillment, recognizing that genuine success is now not measured by way of exterior accolades or achievements, however with the aid of the depth of presence and motive that infuses our day by day endeavors. In the sanctuary of conscious work, we reclaim our inherent ability to thrive amidst the needs and pressures of the current world, embodying a spirit of presence, resilience, and creativity that uplifts and evokes all these round us.

Mindful Parenting

In the sacred experience of parenthood, mindfulness provides a guiding mild amidst the joys and challenges of nurturing the subsequent generation. Through the exercise of aware parenting, we domesticate deeper connections with our children, fostering a nurturing surroundings grounded in presence, compassion, and wisdom.

Being Present with Children: Mindful parenting starts off evolved with a dedication to presence and attunement in our interactions with our children. By slowing down and savoring the valuable moments of every day life, we create opportunities for proper connection and deep bonding with our children. Whether we are playing, reading, or virtually sharing a quiet second together, the exercise of mindfulness invitations us to utterly interact with our children, honoring their special views and experiences with openness and curiosity.

Teaching Mindfulness to the Next Generation: As parents, we have the profound privilege and duty of modeling mindfulness for our children, nurturing their innate ability for presence and self-awareness from an early age. By incorporating easy mindfulness practices into our every day routines, such as conscious breathing, gratitude exercises, or loving-kindness meditations, we provide our teenagers precious equipment for navigating the complexities of their internal and outer worlds with grace and resilience. Moreover, via embodying the characteristics of patience, compassion, and nonjudgmental acceptance in our interactions with our children, we create a nurturing surroundings that fosters their boom and well-being in each factor of their lives.

As we embark on the trip of aware parenting, we find out a profound experience of achievement and connection, recognizing that the best present we can provide our teenagers is the present of our presence and unconditional love. In the sacred area of aware parenting, we sow the seeds of compassion, wisdom, and joy, nurturing the subsequent technology to embody the timeless features of presence, resilience, and kindness that will ripple outwards, shaping the future of our world for generations to come.

{ 4 }

Chapter 4: Overcoming Challenges in Mindfulness Practice

Dealing with Distractions

In the labyrinth of the mind, distractions regularly lurk like shadows, threatening to pull us away from the mild embody of mindfulness. Yet, in the very act of navigating these distractions lies an probability for increase and deepening of our practice. Through the artwork of dealing with distractions, we research to domesticate resilience and presence amidst the ebb and glide of our internal landscape.

Techniques for Refocusing: When distractions inevitably occur all through our practice, we can appoint a range of methods to gently information our interest returned to the current moment. One strategy includes anchoring our recognition in a factor of focus, such as the breath or a precise sensation in the body. By gently redirecting our interest every time it wanders, we instruct the thought to turn out to be extra adept at staying existing amidst the fluctuations of thinking and sensation.

Acceptance of Wandering Thoughts: It's essential to understand that distractions are a herbal section of the human experience, and there is no want to choose or criticize ourselves when our minds wander. Instead, we can domesticate an mind-set of acceptance and nonjudgmental recognition closer to our thoughts, permitting them to come and go like passing clouds in the sky. By embracing the impermanent nature of our internal experiences, we create house for increased peace and equanimity to arise.

As we navigate the terrain of distractions in our mindfulness practice, we find out a profound experience of resilience and internal strength, understanding that each second of presence, no remember how fleeting, brings us one step nearer to the coronary heart of our actual nature. In the dance of interest and distraction, we discover the timeless knowledge that presence is now not a vacation spot to be reached, however a experience to be embraced with open fingers and an open heart.

Managing Resistance and Impatience

In the crucible of mindfulness practice, we frequently come across the bold adversaries of resistance and impatience, lurking in the shadows of our internal landscape, equipped to thwart our efforts and derail our progress. Yet, in the very act of dealing with these challenges head-on lies an possibility for profound boom and transformation. Through the artwork of managing resistance and impatience, we examine to domesticate patience, perseverance, and resilience in the face of adversity.

Embracing Discomfort: When we stumble upon resistance or impatience in our practice, it is tempting to flip away or are seeking for refuge in distraction. However, proper increase happens when we lean into soreness instead than shying away from it. By courageously dealing with the resistance that arises inside us, we create house for recovery and transformation to unfold. Through the exercise of mindfulness, we analyze to preserve house for our soreness with kindness and compassion, recognizing that it is frequently a signal of deeper wounds and unmet wishes in search of our interest and care.

Patience as a Practice: In a world characterized by using instantaneous gratification and regular stimulation, persistence has emerge as a uncommon and valuable commodity. Yet, it is exactly in moments of impatience that the exercise of mindfulness shines most brightly. By cultivating staying power as a practice, we research to embody the unfolding of every second with grace and equanimity, trusting in the knowledge of the existing second to disclose itself in its personal time. Through the mild art of patience, we find out a profound experience of peace and contentment that transcends the stressed striving of the ego, anchoring us in the timeless splendor of the right here and now.

As we navigate the terrain of resistance and impatience in our mindfulness practice, we find out a deep reservoir of internal electricity and resilience that empowers us to face life's challenges with braveness and grace. In the crucible of discomfort, we discover the seeds of transformation, understanding that each and every second of patience, no count number how small, brings us one step nearer to the success of our deepest aspirations and absolute best potential.

Self-Compassion in Difficult Moments

Within the tapestry of our mindfulness practice, there are sure to be moments of warfare and difficulty, when the shadows of doubt and self-judgment loom large. In these moments, the exercise of self-compassion will become a beacon of light, guiding us thru the darkness with gentleness and grace. Through the artwork of self-compassion in hard moments, we analyze to include ourselves with kindness and understanding, fostering a deeper feel of connection and acceptance within.

Being Kind to Oneself: When confronted with challenges or setbacks in our practice, it is all too handy to succumb to the harsh voice of self-criticism and judgment. However, actual recovery takes place when we research to deal with ourselves with the identical kindness and compassion that we would provide to a pricey buddy in need. By cultivating a mild and nurturing internal dialogue, we create a refuge of security and heat inside ourselves, permitting the soft seeds of self-love and acceptance to take root and flourish.

Understanding Impermanence: In the midst of difficulty, it can be tempting to trust that our struggles will closing forever, casting a shadow of hopelessness over our hearts. However, the exercise of mindfulness teaches us to include the impermanent nature of all things, recognizing that even the darkest of clouds will ultimately provide way to the brilliance of the sun. By cultivating an focus of impermanence, we analyze to keep our struggles with a feel of spaciousness and perspective, understanding that they too shall omit in their personal time.

As we navigate the panorama of tough moments in our mindfulness practice, we find out a profound feel of resilience and internal energy that arises from the depths of our being. In the mild include of self-compassion, we discover solace amidst the storms of life, understanding that we are priceless of love and acceptance precisely as we are. With every second of kindness and grasp toward ourselves, we plant seeds of restoration and transformation that ripple outwards, touching the lives of all beings with grace and beauty.

Chapter 5: Cultivating a Lifelong Mindfulness Practice

Establishing a Daily Routine

In the symphony of day by day life, consistency serves as the harmonious melody that weaves mindfulness into the cloth of our existence. Establishing a every day events lays the basis for a lifelong mindfulness practice, nurturing a feel of continuity and integration that permeates each and every thing of our being.

Consistency in Practice: Just as the consistent drip of water wears away stone, so too does the regular exercise of mindfulness progressively sculpt the contours of our minds and hearts. By dedicating time every day to our practice, we create a rhythm of presence and cognizance that infuses our lives with depth and richness. Whether it is a few minutes of meditation upon waking or a aware stroll throughout our lunch break, consistency breeds familiarity and intimacy with the practice, making it an critical phase of our every day experience.

Integrating Mindfulness into Daily Life: Beyond formal exercise sessions, mindfulness invitations us to infuse each and every second of our day with presence and intention. Whether we're washing the dishes, taking walks the dog, or sitting in traffic, each second gives an possibility to domesticate mindfulness and deepen our connection with the current moment. By weaving mindfulness into the material of our every day routines, we radically change the mundane into the sacred, imbuing even the easiest of duties with that means and purpose.

As we commit to organizing a every day movements for our mindfulness practice, we embark on a ride of self-discovery and internal transformation that unfolds with every passing day. In the mild cadence of our each day rituals, we find out a sanctuary of peace and presence, anchoring ourselves in the timeless rhythm of the right here and now.

Cultivating Curiosity and Openness

Within the full-size expanse of the mindfulness journey, cultivating curiosity and openness serves as the compass that courses us thru uncharted territories of the thinking and spirit. Embracing a beginner's mind, we strategy every second with sparkling eyes and an open heart, inviting the ever-unfolding thriller of existence to divulge its wonders in all their splendor.

Embracing a Beginner's Mind: In the tapestry of our day by day experiences, it is convenient to fall into the lure of complacency, assuming that we already comprehend all there is to know. However, the exercise of mindfulness beckons us to shed the boundaries of our preconceptions and biases, adopting a beginner's thinking that is receptive and keen to learn. By coming near every second with a experience of curiosity and wonder, we open ourselves to the endless chances that lie past the confines of our alleviation zone, embarking on a ride of exploration and discovery that is aware of no bounds.

Approaching Practice with Curiosity: In our mindfulness practice, curiosity will become our most depended on ally, guiding us deeper into the recesses of our internal panorama with every breath and each step. Rather than striving to acquire a precise effect or gain a unique goal, we examine to include the method itself with a experience of curiosity and fascination, savoring the nuances and subtleties of our trip as it unfolds in the existing moment. By cultivating an mindset of openness and receptivity closer to some thing arises, we create house for insights and revelations to emerge organically, enriching our exercise with depth and wisdom.

As we domesticate curiosity and openness in our mindfulness practice, we embark on a ride of self-discovery and transformation that transcends the obstacles of the egoic mind. In the boundless expanse of our curiosity, we find out a treasure trove of perception and understanding, unlocking the hidden mysteries of the universe and awakening to the inherent splendor and marvel that permeates each element of our existence.

Nurturing Self-Compassion

Amidst the ebbs and flows of our mindfulness journey, self-compassion emerges as the mild rain that nourishes the seeds of boom and transformation inside us. In moments of subject and self-doubt, we examine to prolong the equal kindness and grasp to ourselves that we would provide to a cherished friend, embracing imperfection as an crucial phase of the human experience.

Kindness Towards Oneself: In a world that frequently needs perfection and achievement, it is handy to fall into the entice of self-criticism and self-judgment. However, the exercise of mindfulness invitations us to domesticate a gentler and greater compassionate relationship with ourselves, recognizing that we are all inherently necessary of love and acceptance, precisely as we are. By extending kindness toward ourselves in moments of combat and suffering, we create a refuge of security and heat within, permitting the smooth seeds of self-love and acceptance to take root and flourish.

Embracing Imperfection: In the crucible of mindfulness practice, imperfection will become our biggest teacher, revealing the hidden splendor and knowledge that lie underneath the floor of our struggles and shortcomings. Rather than striving for an unimaginable best of perfection, we analyze to embody our imperfections with open arms, recognizing them as essential elements of our humanity. By embracing our flaws and vulnerabilities with braveness and humility, we unencumber the transformative electricity of self-compassion, paving the way for restoration and boom to unfold in their very own time.

As we nurture self-compassion in our mindfulness practice, we embark on a ride of profound self-discovery and internal restoration that transcends the boundaries of the egoic mind. In the mild include of self-compassion, we discover solace amidst the storms of life, understanding that we are valuable of love and acceptance precisely as we are. With every second of kindness and appreciation closer to ourselves, we plant seeds of restoration and transformation that ripple outwards, touching the lives of all beings with grace and beauty.

Reflecting on Progress and Insights

Within the tapestry of our mindfulness practice, moments of reflection serve as the mirrors that disclose the depth and splendor of our internal journey. By carving out time for self-reflection and introspection, we create house for boom and perception to flourish, celebrating our growth and honoring the knowledge that arises from within.

Journaling and Self-Reflection: One effective device for cultivating self-awareness and perception is the exercise of journaling. By placing pen to paper and permitting our ideas and emotions to float freely, we reap readability and point of view on the internal workings of our minds and hearts. Whether it is jotting down our ideas after a meditation session or reflecting on our experiences at some point of the day, journaling affords a sacred area for self-expression and self-discovery, illuminating the course to increased grasp and insight.

Celebrating Growth and Insights: In the fast-paced rhythm of contemporary life, it is all too effortless to neglect the growth we've got made on our mindfulness journey. However, by way of taking time to rejoice our increase and insights, we domesticate a experience of gratitude and grasp for the splendor and richness of our experience. Whether it is acknowledging a newfound feel of calm and readability or recognizing the braveness it took to face our internal demons, each step ahead on the course of mindfulness is necessary of social gathering and acknowledgment.

As we mirror on our growth and insights in our mindfulness practice, we deepen our connection to ourselves and the world round us, honoring the timeless knowledge that resides at the core of our being. In the mild include of self-reflection, we find out a sanctuary of peace and presence, anchoring ourselves in the time-less rhythm of the right here and now.

Engaging in Ongoing Learning and Growth

In the boundless expanse of the mindfulness journey, the pursuit of ongoing mastering and boom turns into the compass that publications us toward ever-expanding horizons of grasp and wisdom. By ultimate open to new teachings and practices, we nourish the seeds of curiosity and innovation inside us, cultivating a spirit of lifelong exploration and discovery.

Seeking New Teachings and Practices: The route of mindfulness is wealthy and varied, with infinite teachings and practices ready to be explored. Whether it is attending workshops, analyzing books, or taking part in on line courses, there are infinite possibilities to deepen our appreciation and refine our capabilities on the mindfulness journey. By final open to new teachings and practices, we increase our repertoire of equipment and techniques, enriching our exercise with sparkling insights and views that encourage us to new heights of increase and transformation.

Remaining Open to Growth and Transformation: In the ever-changing landscape of life, boom and transformation are the herbal rhythms that propel us ahead on our trip of awakening. By last open to the winds of exchange and the tides of transformation, we include the inherent impermanence of all things, permitting ourselves to evolve and adapt with grace and resilience. Whether it is confronting our fears, difficult our assumptions, or stepping backyard of our remedy zones, each second of increase brings us one step nearer to the full cognizance of our real potential.

As we interact in ongoing studying and boom in our mindfulness practice, we embark on a trip of self-discovery and internal transformation that transcends the boundaries of the egoic mind. In the boundless expanse of our curiosity and openness, we find out a treasure trove of perception and understanding, unlocking the hidden mysteries of the universe and awakening to the inherent splendor and marvel that permeates each and every thing of our existence.

Conclusion: The Journey Ahead

Reflection on Progress

As we conclude this ride of exploration and discovery, it is crucial to take a second to replicate on the development we've got made alongside the way. Celebrating our achievements, each massive and small, permits us to well known the milestones we've got reached and the increase we've got experienced. By pausing to understand our progress, we domesticate a feel of gratitude and grasp for the efforts we've got invested in our mindfulness practice.

Celebrating Achievements: Each step forward on the mindfulness route is important of celebration. Whether it is studying a new meditation technique, cultivating higher consciousness in day by day life, or experiencing moments of profound insight, each success represents a testimony to our dedication and dedication to growth. By celebrating these milestones, we honor the experience we've got undertaken and the braveness it takes to embark on the route of self-discovery.

Recognizing Growth and Insights: Beyond exterior markers of progress, real increase frequently happens on a deeper, greater refined level. Through moments of introspection and self-reflection, we obtain perception into the workings of our minds and hearts, uncovering hidden patterns and beliefs that structure our ride of the world. By recognizing these insights and integrating them into our lives, we proceed to evolve and make bigger our grasp of ourselves and the world round us.

As we mirror on our progress, we domesticate a experience of self assurance and empowerment that propels us ahead on our mindfulness journey. With every second of reflection, we deepen our connection to ourselves and the world round us, honoring the timeless knowledge that resides inside and embracing the limitless viable that awaits us on the route ahead.

Commitment to Continual Practice

As we stand at the threshold of the experience ahead, it is necessary to reaffirm our dedication to the exercise of mindfulness as a lifelong endeavor. Embracing mindfulness as extra than simply a brief restoration or passing fad, we understand it as a timeless direction of self-discovery and transformation that unfolds with every passing moment. Through unwavering dedication and a steadfast resolve, we domesticate the seeds of mindfulness inside us, nurturing them with care and diligence as they blossom into the radiant plants of awakening.

Embracing Mindfulness as a Lifelong Journey: Mindfulness is now not basically a vacation spot to be reached however instead a experience to be embraced with open palms and an open heart. By recognizing that the direction of mindfulness is one of chronic boom and evolution, we free ourselves from the constraints of perfectionism and achievement, permitting ourselves to ride with curiosity and marvel into the unknown. Embracing mindfulness as a lifelong journey, we open ourselves to the endless probabilities that lie ahead, trusting in the knowledge of the current second to information us on our path.

Cultivating Consistency and Dedication: Like tending to a garden, the practice of mindfulness requires steady care and interest to flourish. By organizing a day by day exercise pursuits and cultivating a feel of self-discipline and dedication, we create the fertile soil in which mindfulness can take root and thrive. Whether it is carving out time for meditation, enticing in conscious motion practices, or really pausing to savor the existing second at some stage in the day, each second of mindfulness contributes to the nourishment of our internal landscape.

As we commit to the chronic exercise of mindfulness, we embark on a trip of self-discovery and transformation that transcends the boundaries of the egoic mind. With every breath, every step, every second of presence, we deepen our connection to ourselves and the world round us, honoring the timeless knowledge that resides inside and embracing the boundless viable that awaits us on the direction ahead.

Embracing Challenges

As we navigate the terrain of the mindfulness journey, it is inevitable that we will stumble upon challenges alongside the way. Yet, instead than viewing these challenges as barriers to be over-come, we can pick out to include them as possibilities for boom and self-discovery. By leaning into the soreness and uncertainty that arises in the face of adversity, we domesticate resilience and perseverance, forging a route of internal electricity and knowledge that leads us ever nearer to the coronary heart of our authentic nature.

Seeing Difficulties as Opportunities for Growth: In the crucible of challenge, we find out the uncooked fabric from which our biggest transformations are born. Whether it is confronting our fears, navigating tough emotions, or dealing with the uncertainties of life, each project we come across provides a threat to deepen our perception of ourselves and the world round us. By embracing these difficulties with braveness and curiosity, we unencumber the hidden gifts they contain, uncovering insights and revelations that propel us ahead on our experience of self-discovery.

Nurturing Resilience and Perseverance: Resilience is now not basically the potential to leap lower back from adversity however as an alternative the capability to thrive in the face of it. By cultivating resilience and perseverance in our mindfulness practice, we advance the internal energy and fortitude to climate life's storms with grace and equanimity. Rather than permitting setbacks to derail us from our path, we use them as stepping stones to increased increase and understanding, trusting in the inherent knowledge of the existing second to information us via even the darkest of times.

As we include challenges on our mindfulness journey, we faucet into a wellspring of internal resilience and braveness that empowers us to face life's uncertainties with grace and resilience. With every impediment we overcome, we deepen our connection to ourselves and the world round us, honoring the timeless knowledge that resides inside and embracing the boundless attainable that awaits us on the direction ahead.

Cultivating Compassion

As we proceed our experience of mindfulness, cultivating compassion will become an imperative cornerstone of our practice. This profound satisfactory of coronary heart and idea now not solely enriches our relationship with ourselves however additionally extends outward, fostering connections and appreciation with all beings. Through the mild artwork of compassion, we create a sanctuary of kindness and warmness within, nurturing the seeds of love and acceptance that stay at the core of our being.

Extending Kindness Towards Oneself and Others: Compassion starts with ourselves. In the busyness of present day life, it is effortless to neglect our very own wants and struggles, however real recovery happens when we research to deal with ourselves with the identical kindness and grasp that we would provide to a pricey pal in need. By extending compassion closer to ourselves in moments of situation and self-doubt, we create a refuge of security and acceptance within, permitting the gentle seeds of self-love and self-compassion to take root and flourish.

Fostering Connections and Understanding: Beyond the boundaries of the self, compassion extends outward, embracing all beings with love and understanding. Through the exercise of mindfulness, we advance the capability to see past the floor of appearances, recognizing the inherent dignity and really worth of each residing being. By cultivating compassion in our interactions with others, we foster deeper connections and understanding, bridging the divides of separation and fostering a experience of cohesion and belonging that transcends the obstacles of the egoic mind.

As we domesticate compassion in our mindfulness practice, we embark on a experience of profound self-discovery and internal transformation that reverberates at some stage in the tapestry of our lives. With every second of kindness and appreciation closer to ourselves and others, we sow seeds of recovery and wholeness that ripple outwards, touching the lives of all beings with grace and beauty.

Integration into Daily Life

As we conclude our exploration of mindfulness, the genuine essence of our exercise lies in its integration into our every day lives. It is no longer adequate to confine mindfulness to formal exercise sessions; rather, we should attempt to weave its standards and teachings into the very material of our existence. Through this integration, we radically change our normal moments into incredible possibilities for growth, presence, and connection.

Weaving Mindfulness into Everyday Routines: Mindfulness is no longer a separate endeavor reserved for extraordinary occasions; it is a way of being that infuses each element of our lives with presence and intention. Whether we're ingesting a meal, on foot in nature, or attractive in dialog with a cherished one, each second gives an possibility to domesticate mindfulness and deepen our connection to the current moment. By infusing our every day routines with mindfulness, we seriously change the mundane into the sacred, awakening to the richness and splendor that surrounds us in each moment.

Embracing the Present Moment in All Its Richness: At its core, mindfulness is about embracing the current second in all its richness and complexity. Rather than getting lost in regrets about the previous or concerns about the future, we examine to anchor ourselves in the right here and now, savoring the sights, sounds, and sensations of the current second with open-hearted awareness. By cultivating this presence, we unencumber the door to a deeper experience of achievement and pleasure that transcends the fleeting pleasures of the external world.

As we combine mindfulness into our every day lives, we embark on a experience of profound transformation and awakening that reverberates in the course of the tapestry of our existence. With every breath, every step, every second of presence, we deepen our connection to ourselves and the world round us, honoring the timeless knowledge that resides inside and embracing the boundless doable that awaits us on the direction ahead.